YOU *CAN* BEAT PERIOD PAIN

Born in Wales and a graduate of the Universities of Kent and Sydney, **Liz Kelly** has written for a range of publications, including *Reader's Digest*, *Cosmopolitan* and *Family Circle*, and now works for *Woman's Day* magazine. She has a special interest in health, education, parenting and women's issues.

YOU *CAN* BEAT PERIOD PAIN

LIZ KELLY

ROBINSON
London

Robinson Publishing Ltd
7 Kensington Church Court
London W8 4SP

First published in Great Britain by
Robinson Publishing Ltd 1995

Published in Australia by
Gore & Osment Publications Pty Ltd

Copyright © Liz Kelly 1992
Copyright © Gore & Osment Publications Pty Ltd

ISBN 1-85487-381-4

All rights reserved. This book is sold subject to the condition that it shall not, by way of trade or otherwise, be lent, re-sold, hired out or otherwise circulated in any form of binding or cover other than that in which it is published and without a similar condition including this condition being imposed on the subsequent purchaser.

A copy of the British Library Cataloguing in Publication Data is available from the British Library

Note
This book is not a substitute for your doctor's or health professional's advice, and the publishers and author cannot accept liability from action as a result of the material in this book. Before commencing any health treatment, always consult your doctor.

Printed and bound in the EC

Contents

Introduction   vii

1 **Bits and Pieces: You and Your Reproductive System**   1
Uterus – fallopian tubes – ovaries – cervix – vagina – vulva – hormones.

2 **Your Periods: What Are They?**   8
Menarche to menopause – myths and magic – the menstrual cycle – what the hormones do – ovulation – what's normal, what's not.

3 **Period Pains: Who Gets Them?**   15
Overcoming prejudice and misunderstanding – family ties – common symptoms – primary dysmenorrhoea (spasmodic dysmenorrhoea) – secondary dysmenorrhoea (congestive dysmenorrhoea) – diagnosing the problem.

4 **Period Pains: What Can Be Done to Help**   22
Treatment of primary dysmenorrhoea – hormone therapy – anti-prostaglandins – analgesics – TENS – surgery – counselling – what you can do yourself – stretching exercises – alternative therapies – treatment of secondary dysmenorrhoea.

5 Premenstrual Syndrome: The Problems of PMS — 35
What is PMS? – who gets it? – what are the symptoms? – what causes it?

6 PMS: What Can Be Done to Help — 40
Progesterone – the pill – Bromocriptine (Parlodel) – anti-depressants – diuretics – vitamin B6 – evening primrose oil – counselling – alternative medicine – what you can do yourself – stressbuster exercises.

7 All About Endometriosis — 53
What causes it? – who gets it? – the symptoms – diagnosis – what can be done to help – hormone therapy – Danazol – oral progesterone – the pill – surgery – natural alternatives – self-help.

8 Too Little, Too Much, Too Late: Or Not at All — 65
Other period problems and their treatments: amenorrhoea (failure to bleed) – menorrhagia (heavy bleeding) – oligomenorrhoea (infrequent, irregular periods) – hypomenorrhoea (light, scanty periods).

9 When the System Goes Wrong — 72
Other problems that can affect a woman's reproductive system – cervical 'erosion' – cervical cancer – uterine or endometrial cancer – polyps – fibroids – ovarian cysts – ovarian cancer – other cancers – the importance of cervical smears.

Helpful Addresses — 77

Glossary — 81

Introduction

There's a line in an old song that says 'Nobody knows the trouble I've seen' and if you're a woman with menstrual problems, that could very well apply to half the world's population – the male half. The key lies in a woman's complex reproductive system. While males and females all have such organs as hearts, lungs, kidneys and so on, the male reproductive system is relatively simple and free of problems.

A woman's, on the other hand, is an intricate arrangement of organs, tubes, glands and hormones. It only needs one thing to be out of balance to upset this complicated pattern and make a woman's life anything from simply uncomfortable to a raging hell 12 or 13 times a year.

Perhaps it's no wonder, then, that so many women describe menstruation as 'the curse'. In the past, those who sought help for painful periods or other distressing symptoms were often told 'it's all in the mind', or 'it's a woman's lot' and that 'what can't be cured must be endured'.

Happily, today, that's no longer the case. New drugs, new techniques and new ways of looking at old remedies mean that for many women, the monthly miseries can be a thing of the past.

Chapter 1
Bits and Pieces
You and Your Reproductive System

The parts of your body that make you a woman are many and varied and aren't always very obvious. Some, like breasts, are easy to see; others are deep inside your brain. The majority, though, are located in the area between the hips known as the pelvic girdle. Here's a quick tour.

UTERUS

At the centre of things is your **uterus** or **womb**. Normally hollow and about the size and shape of a small pear, its muscular walls help it to expand to about the size of a prize watermelon – or even bigger – in pregnancy. The same muscles play a vital role in pushing a baby out into the world during childbirth, but are also linked to the cramps we call period pains. Leading off the wide end of the pear shape are your **Fallopian tubes**, while at the narrow end are the cervical canal and the cervix, also known as the neck of the womb.

The lining of the uterus is known as the

endometrium. It's controlled by the female hormones **oestrogen** and **progesterone** and gets ready each month to receive a fertilised egg. If none arrives, it is shed – forming your monthly bleed.

In most women, the uterus tips forward and rests over your bladder (that's why a very full bladder helps to get a clearer picture of your uterus during an ultrasound examination). But in around 20 per cent of women, it tips backwards to rest against the bowel. This is known as a **retroverted uterus**.

FALLOPIAN TUBES

These two tubes, each about 10–12cm long, are the link between your uterus and your ovaries. The free end of the tubes have delicate fronds which waft in the egg after it leaves the ovary (ovulation). The egg then starts a three-day journey down the tube to the uterus. If on the way it joins up with a friendly sperm, fertilisation takes place.

OVARIES

About the size of a walnut in the shell, the ovaries nestle in the curve of your Fallopian tubes. Although small, they're positive powerhouses as far as your reproductive system is concerned. Not only do they produce the two female hormones oestrogen and progesterone, they also contain hundreds of thousands of eggs – each!

CERVIX

This is the entrance to the uterus. The actual opening is called the cervical os and is normally less than 2mm across but, during childbirth, widens (dilates) to allow the baby to pass through. The cervix also produces a special type of mucus that helps the sperm to pass into the uterus. Some women look for this mucus as a sign that they have ovulated.

> ### FACT FILE
>
> In 16th century Britain, the fertility problems of the house of Tudor changed the course of history. Henry VIII divorced his first wife Katherine because she could not bear him a son. This led to his split with the Catholic church and the establishment of the Anglican church. Despite eventually having six wives, Henry only sired three children – Edward, who succeeded him as king but died young; Katherine's daughter, Mary, who became Queen after Edward and, despite marriage to the lusty Philip of Spain, remained childless because of amenorrhoea; and Elizabeth I, the Virgin Queen, who is thought to have had very irregular periods.

VAGINA

This is the pathway from the cervix to the outside. The walls of the vagina are soft but very muscular, so that it can expand to fit whatever comes its way – a tampon, a penis, a medical instrument, or a baby. It's also the site of the famous G-spot, said to be a woman's most erogenous zone – although no one has been able to pinpoint just where it is!

VULVA

Possibly the sexiest part of your anatomy! The vulva includes both the labia majora or outer lips, which are covered with pubic hair, and the labia minora, which surround the entrance to the vagina. Every woman is different, and your labia minora may be any shade from pale pink to dark brown, as smooth as silk or rather wrinkly, quite small or large enough to protrude below the outer lips.

FACT FILE

Eight weeks before birth, the ovaries of a baby girl contain a staggering seven million seed cells. By the time she is born, that number has dropped to one million, and by the time she reaches puberty, only an estimated 300,000 remain.

BITS AND PIECES

Just below where the labia minora meets is what may be the most sensitive spot in your whole body – your **clitoris**.

Stimulating this little pinkish knob, during intercourse or at other times, can happily bring you to orgasm.

Below the clitoris are both the opening to your urinary tract – the urethra – and the entrance to your vagina. The vaginal opening is surrounded by a soft membrane known as the hymen. This is intact in most – but not all – virgins, but penetration is usually painless.

Female Organs

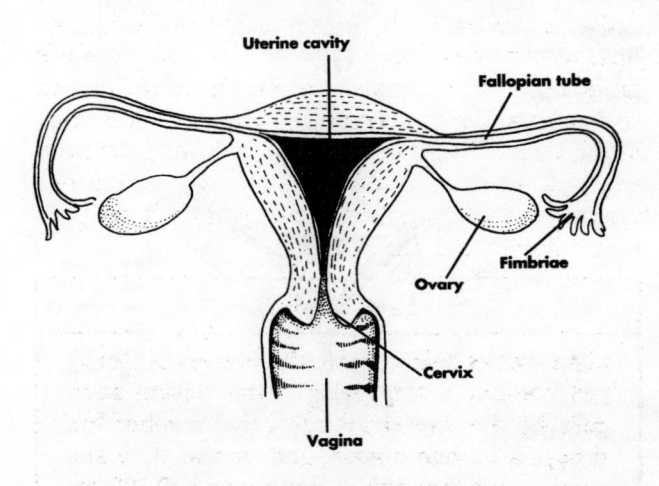

6 YOU *CAN* BEAT PERIOD PAIN

What Happens During Menstruation

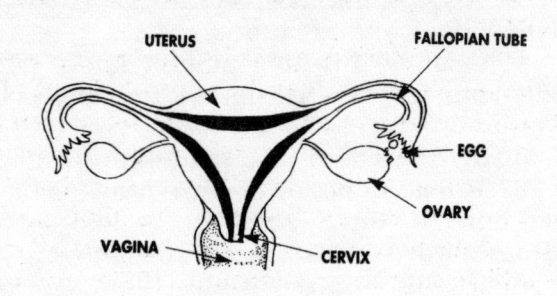

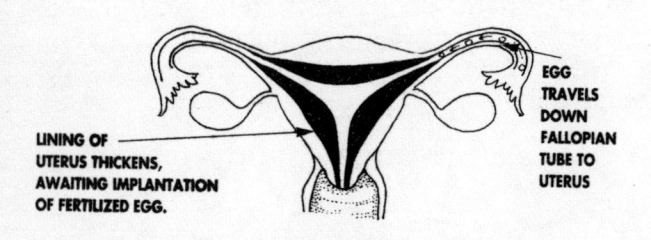

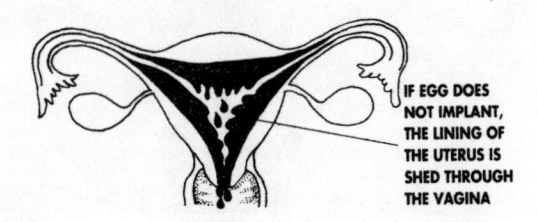

HORMONES

These are the body's chemical messengers and the keys to the whole reproductive system. The two main hormone producers are the ovaries and the **pituitary gland**, and they work in tandem.

Your pituitary gland is located at the base of the brain, and is under the control of part of the brain known as the **hypothalamus**, which also deals with such things as hunger, thirst and body temperature. The pituitary gland releases a range of hormones into the bloodstream, including two linked to your menstrual cycle – follicle stimulating hormone (FSH) and luteinising hormone (LH). These switch on the ovary's production of oestrogen, control the release of the egg, prepare the uterus to receive a fertilised egg, and prompt production of progesterone.

Chapter 2
Your Periods
What Are They?

From adolescence onwards, periods – or the lack of them – are a major feature of any woman's life. From the time of your first menstrual bleed – known as the **menarche** – to the time of your last – the **menopause** – they signal the end of one menstrual cycle and the start of another.

MENARCHE TO MENOPAUSE

In centuries gone by, the average age for a girl to get her first period was around 15, and at this point she was generally regarded as ready for marriage and motherhood.

Today, just as both men and women are getting taller and living longer as a result of better health and improved nutrition, the average age for the menarche is around 13 – and falling. Some girls start menstruating even before they hit their teens; others, especially if they're keen athletes, may not start until they are 16 or 17.

At the same time, and for much the same reason, women today are experiencing menopause later than ever before. In fact, in previous centuries, a woman's lifespan was so short that it was probably a 50-50 chance whether she reached menopause or died first. But in the 1990s, the average age is between 45 and 50.

MYTHS AND MAGIC

While for you periods may be just another part of life, there are many myths, beliefs and rituals associated with them. In some cultures, menstruating women are thought to have special powers – some good, some bad.

In parts of Africa, women have to live in separate women's huts during their periods. Some Aboriginal customs have also required women to live apart during menstruation, while in some New Guinea communities, physical contact with a woman during her period or with menstrual blood is believed to mean slow death for a man.

According to the Roman historian Pliny, menstruating women had the power to turn new wine sour, to make seeds dry up, to cause fruit to fall from trees and bees to die in their hives. They could also blunt the edge of steel – a pretty scary proposition for a soldier about to go into battle in those days – and turn iron and bronze rusty.

On the other hand, menstrual blood could

keep away storms and whirlwinds, and a menstruating woman could cure a whole range of ailments including boils, abscesses and scrofula (a form of tuberculosis)!

More modern myths include that a perm won't take if you're having your period, and that you shouldn't swim, bathe or wash your hair at this time.

> **RELIGIOUS RITES**
>
> The Book of Leviticus in the Bible says a woman is unclean for seven days after the start of her period, and that a man will be contaminated if he lies with her during this time. The Talmud, an important set of laws for Orthodox Jews, forbids intercourse during a woman's period and says that before she can have sex again, she must undergo ritual cleansing in a special bath on the seventh day after the start of her period.

THE MENSTRUAL CYCLE

Each time you start your period, you start a new menstrual cycle. This cycle can be divided roughly into two phases – the time before ovulation and the time after.

The process leading up to ovulation begins with the release of follicle stimulating hormone (FSH) from the pituitary gland. This tells the ovaries to produce oestrogen. When the egg is ready, the ovary sends a message to the pituitary gland to switch to luteinising hormone (LH), which causes the egg to be released – ovulation.

As the egg is busily making its way down the Fallopian tubes and into the uterus, the follicle it left behind develops into what is called the corpus luteum. This produces another hormone, progesterone, along with some oestrogen.

Unless you have conceived in this cycle, the corpus luteum diminishes between 12 and 16 days after ovulation, and the lining of the womb (the endometrium) begins to break down and is shed, in the form of blood, through the cervix and out through the vagina. This is your period. At the same time, your body tells the pituitary gland that your oestrogen levels are low – and the cycle starts again.

FRENCH TALE

In parts of France, it's believed that a woman cannot make curdle-free mayonnaise while she's having her period.

Finnish folklore says she can't churn butter, either.

WHAT THE HORMONES DO

As its name suggests, FSH stimulates the development of egg follicles in one of the ovaries – they usually take it in turns and usually only one egg is ready at a time. (When more than one egg is ready at the same time, there's the possibility of non-identical twins . . . or triplets or . . .)

LH is the chemical messenger that triggers the release of the egg from the follicle.

Oestrogen causes the endometrium to grow and the cervix to produce mucus in readiness for ovulation, the arrival of sperm and – the body hopes – conception.

Progesterone gets the body ready for pregnancy by thickening the cervical mucus, and preparing the endometrium to receive a fertilised egg.

OVULATION

Ovulation is when the mature egg bursts out of its follicle and exits the ovary. It's at this point in your cycle that you can become pregnant, and if you normally bleed every four weeks, it's about midway between the start of your periods.

If you want to conceive or are using natural methods of birth control, you can look for physical signs that ovulation has taken place, including a slight rise in body temperature and a change in your cervical mucus.

Occasionally, you may notice spotting or slight breakthrough bleeding at ovulation. Some women also feel either a dull ache or a sharp pinging pain – this is called mittelschmerz.

> **HOW MANY PERIODS?**
>
> If the average woman starts her periods at 13 and continues until menopause at the age of 48, that's 35 years of periods. If her period arrives every 28 days — or 13 times a year — that's 35 × 13 = 455! Of course, if she has children she'll miss some of those periods — and she'll miss even more if she breastfeeds.

WHAT'S NORMAL, WHAT'S NOT

Unless they're pregnant or suffering certain conditions, most women bleed every month. The average cycle is 28 days, and some women can predict almost to the minute when their period will arrive.

But just as every woman is individual, so is her menstrual cycle, and anything from 21 to 35 days between bleeds is normal, too – provided the length between periods remains much the same for each cycle.

However, if you normally start your period every four weeks or so and then have one that

14 YOU CAN BEAT PERIOD PAIN

is a week or more late, it could in fact be an early miscarriage – and it's worth having a check-up to make sure everything is OK.

Chapter 3
Period Pains
Who Gets Them?

For most women, the menstrual stage – her childbearing time – can last anything from 30 to 40 years. That's a big slice out of anyone's life – especially if you're one of the many women who have period pains (**dysmenorrhoea**).

Depending on their nature, period pains can affect any woman from her early teens to her 30s and 40s. In fact, four out of every five British women suffer at one stage or other.

For some, it may be a bit of discomfort that can be ignored or eased fairly simply. For others, it's an agony that puts them out of action for two, three or four days each month.

In fact, studies indicate that about a third of young adult women need to take time off every now and then because of period pain and, in the US, it's estimated that dysmenorrhoea is to blame for 140 million lost working hours a year.

Many of us, though, just think we have to 'soldier on' – perhaps because we're reluctant to let our colleagues or teachers know what's going on with our bodies; maybe we can't afford to take the time off or fear it will harm our employment prospects or career chances; maybe, if we have young children or other commitments at home, simply because there's no one to take over.

In a way, it's our silent suffering that makes it hard to know how many women are affected – and keeps other women suffering silently, too, because they think they'll be regarded as whingers or shirkers if they take things easy at 'this time of the month' – or because they believe it's just part of 'a woman's lot'.

For many years, that was the typical medical response to period pains, too. Women were often told it was 'all in the mind'. And it wasn't until the 1930s that scientists first noticed that women with anovulatory cycles – cycles in which no egg is released – do not get period pain. This fact alone finally knocked on the head the 'all in the mind' theory.

FAMILY TIES

Some women believe that period pain runs in families – 'Mum has it badly every month, and Gran says she did, too.'

Doctors aren't sure why this is the case. Maybe some women do carry a gene for period pains – but it could also be the case of a mother unwittingly preparing her young daughter to expect to have a bad time, because she did.

TAKE TWO

Although it's true that pain is pain is pain, there are actually two different types of dysmenorrhoea. They're known as **primary** and **secondary dysmenorrhoea**, and their characteristics vary.

COMMON SYMPTOMS

The symptoms of dysmenorrhoea can vary from woman to woman and from period to period – and on whether you have the primary or secondary type. But the most common are:

- General discomfort in the pelvic area
- Intense pain in the form of cramps
- Pain radiating down into the legs and up into the back
- Fatigue
- Mood changes
- Headaches
- Nausea and/or vomiting
- Diarrhoea

PRIMARY DYSMENORRHOEA (OFTEN CALLED SPASMODIC DYSMENORRHOEA)

Primary dysmenorrhoea usually begins early on in your menstrual life, once you start ovulating with each cycle. The pains and other problems start around about the time the bleeding starts and are much the same each month. Some women find that the symptoms ease after they have had a baby – but others find they get worse.

The main culprit in primary dysmenorrhoea is chemical – tiny little molecules called **prostaglandins**, manufactured by the body itself. Among their many roles, prostaglandins affect the widening and narrowing of blood vessels and the tone of muscles you can't exercise yourself – such as the uterus.

They are released to help the uterus to shed its lining, the endometrium, at the end of your

PELVIC INFLAMMATORY DISEASE

Pelvic inflammatory disease (PID) is caused by a number of bacteria, including some transmitted by sexual intercourse, and the risk of getting it increases with the number of sexual partners you have.

There's also a possibility of getting PID after having an IUD fitted — as a result of the germs introduced into your uterus during the process. The risk is highest in the first 20 days after insertion, and recent research suggests the risk can be reduced by taking antibiotics as a precaution.

With PID, you may feel generally unwell, tired, feverish, and off your food; you may have pain in the lower part of your abdomen, backache, and a vaginal discharge.

menstrual cycle, and encourage it to squeeze to clear out its contents. The result is cramps. At the same time, prostaglandins also affect the blood supply in the uterus, causing throbbing.

In general, the thicker the lining of your womb, the heavier your period will be – and the more pain you may get. But this isn't always the case, and it's also a fact that everyone differs in their perception and tolerance of pain.

So the amount of pain you feel may not necessarily relate to the amount of prostaglandins produced by your body or the amount of cramping you suffer.

> The symptoms of an acute attack are obvious, but low-grade infections can smoulder on for months or even years. The big danger here is that PID can lead to infertility because of its effect on the Fallopian tubes; it also increases the risk of an ectopic pregnancy, where the fertilised egg implants outside the uterus, often in one of the Fallopian tubes.
>
> Medical treatment includes antibiotics, painkillers and, in extreme cases, surgery. Heat (such as a hotwater bottle or heating pad) and acupuncture can relieve the symptoms, while natural therapies include garlic to inhibit growth of bacteria; vitamin C; natural antiprostaglandins, such as aspirin; evening primrose oil; and modifying your diet to reduce the amount of saturated fat and increase your intake of fish and raw foods.

SECONDARY DYSMENORRHOEA (OFTEN CALLED CONGESTIVE DYSMENORRHOEA)

Secondary dysmenorrhoea is a different situation altogether. It may often not start until your mid-20s or even later, and rarely clears spontaneously or as a result of pregnancy.

You may get pain or other symptoms only at the time of bleeding or at other times during your cycle, even throughout your cycle. You may also get pain during intercourse – a distressing condition known as **dyspareunia** – or urinary infections.

Unlike primary dysmenorrhoea, which is caused by a normal body function, secondary dysmenorrhoea is a sign that something could be wrong. Its causes are pathological, which means they are linked with disease. These can include:

- Endometriosis (see Chapter 7)
- Pelvic inflammatory disease (PID – see previous page)
- Infection in the Fallopian tubes
- Ovarian cysts (see Chapter 9)
- Fibroids (see Chapter 9)
- Cancers (see Chapter 9)

Secondary dysmenorrhoea can also be traced to:

- Use of an IUD
- Local hormonal imbalance (also sometimes called pelvic congestion syndrome), more likely in premenopausal women

- Congenital abnormalities of uterus and/or the cervix – these are rare, and are generally evident from the time of a woman's first period.

DIAGNOSING THE PROBLEM

When you visit your doctor about period pains, the first thing he or she will do is try to establish whether you have primary or secondary dysmenorrhoea. This is to make sure that you get the appropriate treatment.

The steps are:

- Taking a symptom list and your medical history.
- Carrying out a vaginal pelvic examination – together with your history and symptoms, this may be enough.
- If any disease or abnormality is suspected, the doctor will probably recommend that you have an ultrasound scan.
- Depending on the ultrasound results, a laparoscopy may be required; this is an operation in which the doctor can get a good look at your pelvic cavity and the organs it contains through a laparoscope (a thin instrument a bit like a telescope) inserted through a tiny cut in your abdomen.

Chapter 4
Period Pains
What Can Be Done to Help

Treatment of period pain will differ depending on the cause. With primary dysmenorrhoea, the main aim is either to suppress the pain or the effect of the prostaglandins causing it. With secondary dysmenorrhoea, the focus is usually on eradicating the condition causing the problem.

There is a great range of treatments available, both conventional medical ones and alternative therapies. Some work really well for some women; some work well for many; but none works for every woman – it's just a question of finding which work for you.

PRIMARY DYSMENORRHOEA

There are several types of treatment for this condition, ranging from medication to surgery. They include:

Hormone Therapy

The most common treatment for primary dysmenorrhoea is to put you on the pill. The **combined pill** stops ovulation and so reduces the thickness of the endometrium each cycle, cutting down or even eliminating cramps. The **monophasic pill** (the type that delivers the same amount of oestrogen and progesterone each day) generally works better than the **triphasic** type (in which the hormone levels vary). However, up to 80 per cent of women can expect a reasonably good response whichever pill they take.

The pill's a particularly handy treatment if you also want a contraceptive. But it is a potent drug and there are side effects – such as weight gain, bloating and nausea.

For some women, these outweigh the benefits, so the pros and cons must be explained carefully. Also, if you are trying to get pregnant or don't want to be on the pill for other reasons, this is not the option for you.

An alternative can be to take progesterone for a number of days in the second part of the cycle, especially if you have heavy periods. This is usually in tablet form.

Another hormonal remedy – although rarely – used is drugs that mimic the effect of adrenalin. These are called beta-sympathomimetics, such as Ventolin or Bricanyl. They relax muscles and are more generally used to ease asthma attacks, but because they also affect the uterus they are useful in efforts to halt premature labour. The problem is that they do not work all that well for period pain, and the side effects – rapid heartbeat, palpitations and feelings of anxiety – can be very distressing.

Anti-prostaglandins

These drugs block the production and action of the prostaglandins, and can be effective in 80 to 90 per cent of women. The most common medications in this group are Ponstan and Naprosyn.

Apart from the fact that they are not contraceptives, the big advantage that anti-prostaglandins have over the pill is that they only need to be taken at the very first sign that your period is starting – whether that's the first trace of blood or the first cramp. Some women need more than others, and you and your doctor will have to experiment a bit to find the best dose for you.

There are side effects too, and anti-prostaglandins are not recommended for women with certain medical problems, such as stomach ulcers and kidney problems, except occasionally in the short term. They can also irritate the stomach, causing gastro-intestinal upsets.

Analgesics

Painkillers, especially those containing codeine, may also work. Some of these may be available on prescription only, but the over-the-counter types containing aspirin and paracetamol may be sufficient for you. Aspirin can work especially well because it also has an anti-prostaglandin effect – but it can also irritate the stomach.

TENS

Some women report a dramatic improvement with the use of a treatment called TENS – transcutaneous electrical nerve stimulation. This works by providing a light electrical current across the skin, stimulating the nerve endings which in turn block messages to the brain about pain perception. TENS machines are often used in specialist pain clinics and some physiotherapy centres and can be effective in up to 50 per cent of women whose period pain has not responded well to other treatments.

DEEP BREATHING

Stand with your feet apart and arms by your side and breathe in deeply, filling your lungs; when they are full, start to breathe out slowly and evenly through your nose; when your lungs feel empty, lift your shoulders and bring your arms forward in front of your chest as if to squeeze out any remaining air. Do this several times until you feel relaxed.

Surgery

Few doctors these days recommend surgery, although for some older women with very severe dysmenorrhoea, a hysterectomy may be suggested. There is also an operation known as a pre-sacral neurectomy, in which nerves going into the uterus are divided – but this is not common.

At one time it was believed that period pains were the result of the cervix being too tight, so a D&C (dilation and curettage) was used to reduce the discomfort. But this 'solution' is not widely used today and, in any case, gives only temporary relief.

Counselling

Unlike in previous decades when doctors often dismissed a woman's distress over period pains by telling her 'it's all in the mind' or that 'it's a woman's lot', many doctors today offer counselling and advice. Reassurance, plus suggestions for self-help and lifestyle adjustments around your period pain, help many women.

WHAT YOU CAN DO

For various reasons, not every woman will want to consult a doctor about period pains, especially if they do not interfere too much with her life – and there are many ways that you can help yourself when they do strike.

- **Painkillers:** Simple, over the-counter analgesics are readily available and are probably the most common home remedy.
- **Heat:** Holding a hotwater bottle or a heating pad against your tummy is also fairly popular. So is a lovely hot bath – throw in some herbs or aromatic oil for a relaxing effect.
- **Hot drinks:** A good cup of tea or coffee can make you feel better; or try ginger tea (see box, below). Other herbal teas such as mint can also help to ease abdominal pain, especially if you feel the need to burp – fresh mint is best, or look for dried peppermint in your health food shop.
- **Herbal remedies:** Many of the companies that sell vitamin and mineral supplements offer a range of products containing angelica (dong quai) and based on an ancient Chinese herbal combination, designed to ease menstrual problems. Vitamin B6 and evening primrose oil can also be effective.

GINGER TEA

Take four slices of fresh green ginger and chop finely; pour over a cup of boiling water; cover (to stop the important volatile oils escaping) until cool enough to drink. This is good for any type of cramping pain, and also for nausea and morning sickness.

- **Calcium and magnesium:** Some women have found that taking a combination of calcium and magnesium can help; but this is not a short-term remedy and needs to be taken every day for at least a couple of months before you notice any major effect. Take care not to take more than the recommended dose as too much of these minerals can harm your system.
- **Relaxation:** Because of the changes in their bodies and their hormones, many women find the time of their period particularly stressful, and when we are stressed, our pain often becomes far less bearable. There's a wide variety of techniques available, ranging from exercises to soothe tense muscles to relaxation tapes, meditation, hypnotherapy and so on. But if you're at work or school or at home with young children, you can't always get the opportunity or the time, so some deep breathing exercises may be more convenient. (See box, p.25)
- **Stop smoking:** Your pelvic organs need a good supply of oxygen, and smoking reduces this; in fact, surveys have found that women who smoke heavily are more likely to get more severe or more frequent dysmenorrhoea.
- **Watch your diet:** Make sure you have foods that are high in natural anti-prostaglandins like calcium and magnesium, and the B group vitamins (such as low-fat dairy products, fruit juices, whole foods, raw vegeta-

bles, figs, nuts and seeds); reduce the amount of saturated animal fats and increase your intake of polyunsaturates and fish oils.
- **Exercise:** cycling, walking and swimming are all recommended, as are stretching exercises that help you relax and ease any lower back trouble that may be causing problems with the pelvic nerves and blood supply, leading to congestion.
- **Yoga:** This is a great way to relax the body and the mind; the bow or the cobra poses are especially good (see pp. 30–1).
- **Pelvic rocking:** Bellydancing and exercises of that type can help to relieve pain by relaxing the muscles and improving blood supply in the pelvic area.
- **Massage:** Lightly massaging the back and lower abdomen can do wonders for some women, the theory being that it gives a different message to the sensitive nerve endings in and just below the skin in the area. Do it yourself or, even better, get someone to do it for you.
- **Orgasm:** You may feel too awful to contemplate this but just as getting sexually aroused increases the blood supply to the pelvic area, orgasm can relieve the resulting congestion.

Alternative Therapies

- **Homeopathy:** Homeopaths treat each woman as an individual with an individual problem, and say that no single remedy suits

STRETCHING EXERCISES

These exercises are recommended by the Family Planning Association:

Pelvic press
Lie flat on the floor, face down, palms on the floor beside your shoulders. Push your palms down and raise your head and shoulders off the floor until your arms are outstretched; repeat several times.

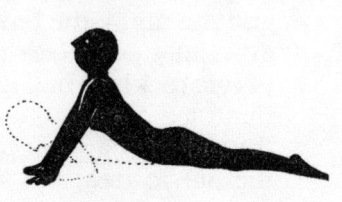

Crouch
Lie on your side, with your knees drawn up to your chest and your head tucked under to touch your knees in the foetal position.

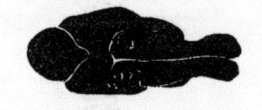

PERIOD PAINS 31

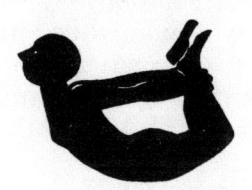

Pelvic rock
Lie flat on the floor, face down. Stretch your arms behind you, arch your back and reach behind to grasp your ankles, bending your knees and bringing your feet up to meet your hands – your legs, head and shoulders should all be off the floor. Gently rock.

Stretching
Stand with your back against the wall, with your head, shoulders, heels and as much of the rest of your body as possible touching the wall. Try to feel as though your head is being drawn upwards, making you as tall as possible. Do this often – it's great for your posture as well as relieving period pain.

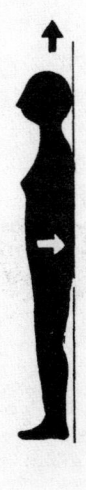

everyone, and different combinations work better for different women. So you should consult a trained practitioner rather than try to treat yourself in this way. Among the more commonly used treatments are vitus agnus castus, the appropriately named crampbark (an old American Indian remedy) and false unicorn root.

- **Acupuncture:** One of the secrets of acupuncture is that it gets the body to release its own natural painkillers – these are called endorphins – which is why it is sometimes used instead of an anaesthetic in surgery or during labour. Some women get great relief through acupuncture and may need only a few sessions; others may need to go more regularly.
- **Chiropractic:** Problems with the lower back can disturb things in the pelvic area, affecting both the blood supply and the nerve

WHAT TO EAT

Calcium — dairy foods (use skim milk or low-fat only), cereals, vegetables and pulses

Magnesium — soy beans, nuts, brown rice, yeast, seafood, bananas, dried fruit, meat and vegetables

Vitamin B — brown rice, nuts, yeast, green vegetables, dairy food, liver, fish, grains, pulses and eggs endings. For some women, sorting out their back trouble can signal an end to dysmenorrhoea.

SECONDARY DYSMENORRHOEA

Because the causes of secondary dysmenorrhoea vary, so do the medical and surgical treatments available. For some women, it can be as simple as removing an IUD or taking a course of antibiotics for PID. For others, it could mean surgery to remove polyps, cysts or fibroids (see Chapter 9) or a combination of surgery and hormone therapy for endometriosis (see Chapter 7). Because of the side effects of treatment – whether by drugs or surgery – for some women, the best therapy may just be to do nothing. You should always discuss all the options carefully with your doctor, asking about side effects and other possible treatments, as the best remedy for you is the one that suits you best – and that could simply mean self-help or other methods to reduce the pain and discomfort of each cycle.

As far as alternative therapies are concerned, you have a big range to choose from – again depending on the cause of the dysmenorrhoea.

Homeopaths treat the whole person not just the disease, so individual consultations are essential to determine the best combination of remedies for you. Some women find great relief in homeopathic remedies for endometriosis and other causes of pain, while others swear by Chinese herbal medicine, massage and acupuncture.

Chapter 5
Premenstrual Syndrome
The Problems of PMS

While most women notice some changes to their body and their emotions prior to the start of their period (some studies suggest over 90 per cent), about one in three of us suffer from significant **premenstrual syndrome (PMS)**.

About 10 per cent suffer to the extent that it is a real problem, perhaps to the point that just about every month they feel their lives and their relationships with their partner, family, friends and at work are being seriously affected.

As with period pains, the true cost of PMS isn't known – either in economic terms because of work time-off lost, or in social terms because of its effect on those around us. But it must be considerable.

WHAT IS PMS?

The first scientific description of PMS came as far back as 1931, but despite many studies since then, doctors today are really no closer to understanding it.

Broadly defined, PMS is a cluster of symptoms which are both physical and psychological, linked to the ebb and flow of the menstrual cycle. An earlier name was PMT – premenstrual tension – but this was dropped as the experts came to realise that there was a lot more involved than simply feeling uptight every month.

Although doctors in ancient Greece described premenstrual changes such as feelings of heaviness, headaches, ringing in the ears and specks before the eyes, PMS seems to be far more common today than in previous times. One reason for that is that women today generally delay childbearing and have fewer or no children – and so more periods. Some researchers also blame the fact that today's general environment is far more toxic than it was in previous centuries.

STRANGE BUT TRUE

Groups of young women living together often find that their periods start to synchronise – and everyone is likely to feel lousy at the same time.

The French have long been known for their crimes of passion, but in the past 10 years or so, PMS has been raised – and sometimes accepted – as a defence in legal cases in the US and the UK.

But it's important to remember that not all changes in the time leading up to your period are PMS. For this reason, it's a good idea to keep a menstrual calendar for at least two months (preferably longer), noting all the physical and psychological or emotional changes. This can help to detect any underlying problems that might be mistaken for PMS.

WHO GETS IT?

Research indicates that women more vulnerable to stress are more liable to suffer severe symptoms. After all, if you're finding it hard to cope anyway or are just keeping your head above water, the impact of body or mood changes over which you seem to have no control can be devastating.

Many women find that the symptoms get worse with age, and studies have also suggested a link between PMS and your chances of suffering postnatal depression.

Women on the pill, however, tend to suffer fewer and shorter symptoms.

WHAT ARE THE SYMPTOMS?

The symptoms can vary; in fact, there are between 150 and 180 of them on the various PMS classification lists. Most are associated with the days following ovulation and leading up to the start of your period – a time known as the **premenstruum**. They include:

- water retention and bloating
- weight gain
- breast tenderness
- headaches
- skin problems
- backache
- changes in bowel habits
- clumsiness or being accident-prone
- mood changes
- tension
- anxiety
- food cravings (normally for sweet things, thought to be linked to hormonal changes and low blood sugar)
- irritability
- depression
- changes in energy levels – usually lethargy and fatigue, although some women have short but intense energy boosts.

WHAT CAUSES IT?

There are almost as many theories about the cause of PMS as there are symptoms. But the most popular at the moment is that it is linked to an imbalance in the body's oestrogen and progesterone levels. Experts such as British researcher Dr Katharina Dalton believe this imbalance affects production of brain chemicals such as serotonin and endorphins, and leads to lower blood sugar.

Other researchers say prostaglandins may be to blame; or that your body is deficient in vital vitamins; or that too much of the hormone prolactin is produced.

Another important theory centres on psychological factors and the impact of stress.

Chapter 6
PMS
What Can Be Done to Help

When someone somewhere comes up with a general cure for PMS, there'll be a fortune to be made. In the meantime, there are almost as many ways of treating the syndrome medically as there are theories about its cause, and to be most effective drug therapy should be based on your specific symptoms.

Two forms of hormone therapy seem to work well for many women with troublesome PMS:

- **Progesterone:** The idea behind the treatment is that by boosting your progesterone level in the second part of your menstrual cycle – the 14 or so days after ovulation known as the luteal phase – a range of PMS symptoms can be eased. These can include mood swings and feelings of irritability and depression, or physical problems such as headaches, food cravings, fluid retention, bloating and weight gain.

  Both natural and synthetic progesterone are available, taken orally, vaginally and, in some cases, by injection or implant. Some doctors prefer to prescribe natural progesterone; others recommend synthetic varieties such as dydrogesterone (Duphaston), which closely resembles the hormone your own body produces.

The initial treatment is usually for three months, and the effects – and side effects – are then reviewed. You will have to keep a careful record of your responses. These will vary from woman to woman, and you and your doctor may have to experiment a little with dosage to find the one that works best for you. While many women report a worthwhile easing of symptoms, for some women, however, progesterone brings little benefit.

- **The pill:** Because it delivers a set amount of oestrogen and progesterone through your cycle, the pill not only suppresses ovulation, but also your body's natural hormone fluctuations. This can make a big difference to some PMS sufferers, but for others the pill's side effects – such as nausea, bloating and so on – just make the situation worse.

  Also, as with its use in treating period pain, the pill is a contraceptive and has to be taken throughout your cycle, making it inappropriate for some women.

Other medication may be offered to relieve specific symptoms:

- **Bromocriptine (Parlodel):** This can help to reduce breast soreness. But it offers no relief from the psychological and emotional symptoms of PMS and has side effects including nausea and vomiting.
- **Anti-depressants:** At one stage, these were

DIET AND PMS

A balanced diet with plenty of complex carbohydrate, fresh fruit and vegetables and fibre, a moderate amount of protein but low in sugars and fats will provide you with essential vitamins (including A, B, C and E) and minerals (such as calcium, potassium, magnesium and iron) – all of which play a role in reducing PMS symptoms.

often prescribed to help a woman handle the depression and mood changes of PMS, but are not a common therapy these days. Depending on what is used, anti-depressants have their own problems, including the risk of dependency.

- **Diuretics:** These may offer some relief for water retention, bloating and weight gain but do not always work. Perhaps the most effective is aldactone (spironolactone).
- **Vitamin B6 (pyridoxine):** Some women find their PMS is relieved by boosting their levels of vitamin B6. This plays a part in producing brain chemicals, such as serotonin, which help to regulate our moods. Vitamin B6 can help with PMS headaches, depression, irritability and fatigue. But just because a little does some good, it doesn't mean that a lot will do much better. In its correct dosage – between 50mg and 200mg a day, depending on the individual – it's

fine, but in very large amounts it can have a toxic effect and lead to what's called peripheral neuropathy (tingling and numbness in the hands and feet). So stick to your recommended dose. Other B group vitamins can also help PMS, and some women find that taking a B-complex rather than just B6 brings more benefits.
- **Evening primrose oil:** This is another 'natural' therapy that many doctors are happy to prescribe for PMS, either alone or in combination with other remedies. Evening primrose oil is high in vitamin E and can help to ease headaches, premenstrual aches and pains, depression and water retention.

GOOD TO EAT

- Fresh fruit and vegetables (especially green, leafy vegetables, citrus fruit, bananas, capsicum, garlic, peas, avocado, parsley, figs and dates) for vitamins B1, B3, B6, A, C and E, potassium, magnesium, calcium and zinc.
- Grains, cereals, nuts, pulses and brown rice for complex carbohydrates, vitamins B1, B3, B6; magnesium, zinc and calcium.
- Dairy foods (low-fat) for calcium, vitamins B1, B3, B6; zinc.
- Oils (vegetable oils, such as sunflower and other polyunsaturates) and fish (such as sardines, tuna, etc) or fish oils for vitamins A, E, B1, B6, potassium and iron.

- **Counselling:** This can mean any of a number of things, but having someone like a doctor who is prepared to take your symptoms seriously and to listen to your feelings undoubtedly helps many women. Sometimes, reassurance that it's part of a naturally occurring cycle or just sharing your sad, bad feelings can lift the burden – at least for a while – and discovering the nature of the symptoms will help you, your family and others understand why you turn into an angry, short-fused bundle of misery every three to four weeks.

ALTERNATIVE MEDICINE

As with period pain, different alternative practitioners can offer a range of remedies for various aspects of PMS.

But because there are so many possible symptoms, you really need to discuss your particular ones with your particular therapist. For instance, with homeopathy, each of the symptoms is a clue to what is happening in your body so your homeopath will look at the overall picture and prescribe accordingly.

The result is that your particular remedy could well be a combination of various ones – maybe including evening primrose oil, vitamin B6, trace elements or herbal painkillers such as feverfew tablets or white willow bark

– and may be quite different to the one prescribed by the same person for your friend, sister, mother or daughter who also has PMS.

WHAT YOU CAN DO

For severe PMS, you are probably better off seeing your doctor or, if you prefer, someone who specialises in alternative medicine (some doctors combine these). But if your PMS symptoms are not severe enough to disrupt your life, or only occur sporadically, there are remedies you can try yourself.

- **Vitamin B6:** This occurs naturally in a range of foods or can be taken as a supplement (but take care not to exceed the recommended dose). It's best if taken in a B-complex or as

---

FOOD CRAVINGS

Researchers have also found that women are more likely to suffer food cravings in the second part of their menstrual cycle, because of changes in their blood sugar levels. Of course, cravings like this are never for broccoli or liver or apples – they're for sweet foods such as cakes, biscuits and perhaps the greatest 'comfort' food of all, chocolate. So if you break your diet at this time, blame your hormones.

part of one of the mineral and vitamin combinations specifically designed for women.

- **Check your diet:** Go for a balanced diet high in complex carbohydrates, fresh fruit and vegetables and fibre (see p.43 for details).
- **Limit salt intake:** Sodium is one of the big culprits in water retention, bloating and temporary weight gain, so cut back on the salt in your diet by avoiding processed and takeaway food and reduce its use in cooking or at the table.
- **Painkillers:** Simple analgesics such as paracetamol or aspirin will ease premenstrual headaches and other aches.
- **Check your caffeine intake:** Too much caffeine (in tea, coffee and chocolate) can bring on headaches, whether they're related to PMS or not.
- **Heat:** It's an age-old remedy but a comforting one, whether you opt for a hot bubble bath, a hotwater bottle, a heating pad, a hot drink or just a warm bed.
- **Stop smoking:** On top of its other health risks, smoking also affects your blood supply and this can contribute to pelvic congestion and discomfort.
- **Wear a good bra:** PMS-tender breasts need good support, so even if you generally prefer to go without, get yourself a good bra for this part of your cycle.
- **Loose clothing:** If you feel bloated, uncomfortable or just not your best, put away

those tight jeans, slinky skirts and waist-cinching belts and switch to loose clothing; after all, there's no point in adding to your discomfort with clothing that only emphasises the issue.

STRESS AND PMS

Work by the Key Centre in Melbourne, Australia, indicates that many women with severe PMS often have low self-esteem. They may also be more vulnerable to stress, with a long history of struggling to cope with life and its problems. With PMS come changes over which they have no control — and that can be enough to tip the balance the wrong way. In fact, most women with severe PMS say they can deal with the physical discomforts, but the pain of the negative moods (anger, depression and irritability) and the effect on their families, work and social relationships are very distressing. These women may benefit from learning new coping strategies, with the help of trained psychologists. This involves keeping a daily record of their responses to events and stresses throughout the menstrual cycle, identifying which trigger which reactions, and then 'unlearning' old patterns of behaviour and learning new ones. Another way is teaching women how to be assertive.

- **Massage:** Light fingertip massage of the stomach and back area can help block some of the pain messages to your brain. Try it yourself or, even better, get a friend or your partner to do it – that feeling of being cosseted helps, too.
- **Exercise:** Maintaining your normal exercise routine improves your circulation and helps to relieve feelings of stress. Swimming, walking and cycling are good, and yoga is excellent. You could also try special exercises, designed to relieve stress (see 'Stressbusters' pp. 50–51).
- **Recognise and accept the symptoms as PMS:** Being able to recognise your own cycle of changes will help you to see them as symptoms of PMS, and not signs that you're falling apart. That's especially important with the mental and emotional swings of PMS. So, think about it – and if you notice you're always tired and tetchy in the week or so before your period, accept it as part of your cycle and let your family know, too. Then you can adjust your life to compensate – maybe by cutting back housework (after all, no one ever suffers if the carpets aren't vacuumed or the kitchen windows aren't cleaned, but you do suffer if you insist on martyring yourself to 'carry on as normal') or better still, sharing it out among the family. At work, try making a pile of those routine jobs that you hate and tackle them on the days when you don't have your usual sparkle.

STRESSBUSTERS

You can do the first three sitting down:

Shoulder stretch – With your body straight and chin level, arms loose at your sides, lift one shoulder up until it is as close to your ear as you can manage; hold for a count of 10; drop shoulder. Relax for a count of five, then repeat with other shoulder. Alternate shoulders several times, then finish by lifting both simultaneously, hold for five, drop.

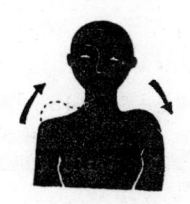

Shoulder circles – With your body straight and arms by your sides, move one shoulder in a complete forward circle; do this three or four times, then reverse direction. Repeat with other shoulder. Finish by moving both shoulders together – four or five times forward, then back.

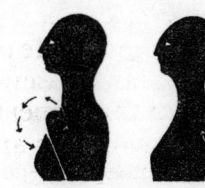

50 YOU CAN BEAT PERIOD PAIN

Chair pushes – Sit on a straight-backed chair with your feet flat, your knees a chairwidth apart, your hands on your thighs just above the knees, fingers spread. Lean forward slightly, raising your shoulders and keeping your back straight. Breathe in deeply, then breathe out through your mouth, emptying your lungs and pulling in your stomach muscles as you do. Hold for a few seconds, then release. Repeat.

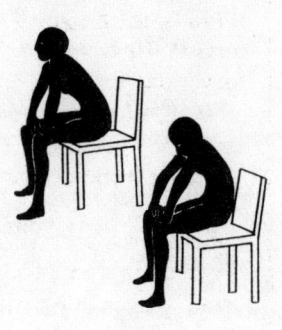

Camel – Start on your hands and knees, palms flat, back straight. Breathe in deeply through your nose, then breathe out slowly through your mouth, pulling your stomach muscles in and up as you arch your back; tuck your head in; hold for 10. Breathe in through your nose, flattening your back and lifting your head as you do until you reach your starting position. Repeat five or six times.

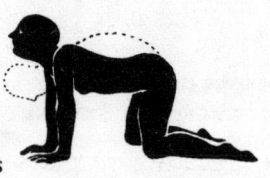

A WORD OF WARNING

PMS is not a sign of weakness, nor is it an indication that women are somehow physically, psychologically or emotionally inferior to men – who, of course, don't get PMS because they don't get periods. (The cynics among us might say that if men did get periods and PMS, there would be a lot more research into causes and treatments and a far greater acceptance of both as subjects to be discussed openly.)

PMS is something that occurs naturally as a woman goes through her menstrual cycle, and not something that needs to be hidden away as a shameful secret. Nor should it be used to justify treating women in the workforce, for instance, any differently to their male colleagues.

Whatever your situation, if PMS is getting you down, it's not a time to try to perform miracles. Switch into a lower gear instead, and leave the miracles until later.

- **Rest:** Accept that you're not feeling great and try to make time for rest and relaxation. Many women, especially those with children or who care for elderly and infirm parents, find this hard – so this is the time to delegate responsibilities or call on family and friends to help.
- **Talk about it:** Don't keep it to yourself. The negative mood changes of PMS can leave you feeling very alone, misunderstood, irritable

or maybe resentful. Your emotions can affect your whole family and even your friends, so discuss your feelings with them. You're likely to find some of them have PMS problems, too. If you feel you can't raise the issue with family or friends, try a professional such as your doctor.

Chapter 7
All About Endometriosis

Research suggests that endometriosis affects between 10 and 15 per cent of women at some stage. But it is impossible to say exactly how many women may have it because some have no symptoms, and others may simply be undiagnosed. However, it is thought to be the second most common condition affecting women during their menstruating years and one of the main causes of secondary dysmenorrhoea.

Many women on IVF (in vitro fertilisation) programmes are there because of endometriosis.

WHAT CAUSES IT?

This condition gets its name from the endometrium (lining of the womb).

As with so many of the conditions related to menstruation, the cause is not clear. However, the most popular theory is that endometriosis occurs when tiny pieces of endometrium find their way into the abdominal area as a kind of backwash through the Fallopian tubes (retrograde menstruation). There, they implant on other organs. Endometriosis is most usually found on the ovaries, the tubes and the outside of the uterus, and, occasionally, on the bladder or the bowel. In very rare cases, it may even be found in the lungs and other body organs.

The implants can be the size of a pinhead or a large cyst. They respond to the cyclic production of hormones, growing and bleeding with each cycle.

But there is nowhere for the blood to go, and the result is congestion, pain and the formation of scar tissue (adhesions) which can block the Fallopian tubes or cause organs to stick together.

VISUALISATION

This technique helps you to use mind images to blot out pain. For instance, you could picture yourself lying on a secluded beach, with the sun warming your skin, the breeze gently swaying the trees and the waves breaking softly on the golden sands. Or you could 'pack' your endometriosis into a suitcase and send it far away. Some people prefer to visualise the endometrical implants being destroyed by your body's natural defence system.

WHO GETS IT?

After it was first accurately described by an American doctor back in 1931, many doctors regarded endometriosis as 'the career woman's disease'. That's because for many years it was most frequently diagnosed in white, middle-class, career-oriented women in their 30s and early 40s who had delayed childbearing to get on in their jobs and whose endometriosis was only diagnosed when they had problems getting pregnant.

But the truth is very different. Today, following the development of ultrasound and laparoscopy, it is known to be present in all types of women, of all ages, races, and inclinations.

There's speculation that endometriosis is on the increase; but some experts believe that it's more the case that an increasing number of doctors today are aware of its existence and that more women are less likely to put up with its symptoms – and that, as a result, it's simply being diagnosed more.

THE SYMPTOMS

These can vary from nothing to:
- painful periods
- pain on intercourse (dyspareunia)
- lower abdominal aching
- sciatica
- backache
- tiredness
- infertility

DIAGNOSIS

There is no easy way to diagnose endometriosis. In fact, although doctors may suspect it, the only accurate diagnosis is visual – by detecting its presence through laparoscopy. Early diagnosis is vital, as endemetriosis is thought to get worse the longer it remains untreated.

Unfortunately, the early symptoms can be hard to pinpoint and there are still doctors who refuse to take women's complaints about pain seriously, especially if they are teenagers or under the age of 25. So they may find themselves going back to the doctor year after year – or from doctor to doctor – seeking explanations and relief. In fact, a survey by the Endometriosis Association in Victoria, Australia, has found that the average time between the start of symptoms and diagnosis is more than six years. Also, the younger you are, the less likely that endometriosis will be suggested as a cause of your pains. So it's definitely worthwhile shopping around to find a doctor who is aware and supportive.

WHAT CAN BE DONE TO HELP

If endometriosis is diagnosed, the big question that you and your doctor will have to consider is what to do about it.

Conventional treatment can vary from doing nothing (except observe) to drug therapy or even surgery. Bearing in mind that, in some women, endometriosis is only detected by chance as a result of surgery for some other condition in the pelvic area and that the measures taken to alleviate it can be either potent or permanent, a lot will depend on the effect that it is actually having on you.

The main types of treatment are hormone therapy, designed to eradicate the endometriosis, or symptomatic, designed to relieve the symptoms.

DYSPAREUNIA

If sex causes you pain, the results can be devastating. Not only is pain a great turn-off for you, it may also turn your partner off too — because he doesn't want to hurt you. In addition, it can also be a big blow to a woman's self-image and, of course, it makes it difficult if you want to get pregnant. The key is good communication with your partner. Talk about the problem; explore other ways of showing your love for each other; experiment with different positions and angles of penetration to find the ones that cause you the least discomfort.

Hormone Therapy Includes:

- **Danazol:** Danazol (Danol) is actually a weakened form of the male hormone testosterone. Taken daily, it acts on the pituitary gland to turn off production of female hormones, suppressing ovulation. With the ebb and flow of the menstrual cycle at an end, the endometrial implants can become inactive and then shrink and die. The average length of a course of treatment is six months but you should notice some improvement as early as four weeks. Up to 80 per cent of women report complete or partial relief, but of these about a quarter find their symptoms recur.

The big drawback is the side effects and there's no way of predicting how you will respond. Some women say they've never felt better; some find the side effects bearable; but for others, they are intolerable. The most common include weight gain, fluid retention, bad skin, greasy hair, reduced breast size, an increase in body and facial hair, deepening of the voice and even enlargement of the clitoris. There can also be the type of symptoms more commonly associated with menopause – hot flushes, night sweats and vaginal dryness. Because of risk to the foetus, Danazol's manufacturers recommend that you take precautions to avoid conceiving while on this potent drug.

- **Oral progesterone:** Dydrogesterone (Duphaston) has been used in Britain for a quarter of a century, and seems particularly effective in early cases. Compared to other drugs, the side effects are relatively minor and include breast tenderness, bloating, weight gain, headache, fatigue, nausea and cramps – most of which disappear with time.

Other, stronger types of progesterone are also available. They include Provera and its long-acting injectable form Depo-Provera, and Primolut N. Like Duphaston, no one's quite sure how these synthetic progesterones work on the endometriosis, only that they can provide significant relief for a number of women. Side effects can include weight gain, bloating, tiredness, nausea, bleeding and loss of libido.

INFERTILITY

Endometriosis is one of the most common causes of infertility among women over the age of 25, and it's estimated that between 30 and 40 per cent of women with endometriosis are infertile. The main reasons seem to be adhesions blocking the Fallopian tubes, or hindering the expulsion of the egg from the ovaries. The good news is that about half the women affected do eventually conceive.

- The pill: Once thought a good option, the pill is now regarded as a less effective treatment. However, some doctors believe long-term use may slow down progression of the disease. Side effects include bloating, fluid retention, nausea, headaches, depression, skin problems, changed libido and a greater tendency to thrush.

- A number of drugs known as GnRH (gonadotropin releasing hormone) or LHRH (luteinising hormone releasing hormone) agonists are currently being trialed. These are designed to stop the pituitary gland sending chemical messengers to the ovaries, cutting off production of oestrogen and progesterone (without which menstruation cannot occur) – rather like turning the power off at the sub-station. The side effects are the same as those caused by low oestrogen at menopause.

PREGNANCY

At one stage, doctors believed that pregnancy could cure endometriosis because it puts an end – for nine months at least – to a woman's normal hormonal changes. The theory was that during this time, the endometrial implants would shrivel up and die, possibly never to recur. Alas, research does not bear this out. The truth seems to be that while pregnancy may alleviate the problem for a while, it is very likely to return.

- **Surgery:** If drug therapy doesn't help, surgery may be another option, either on its own or in combination with medication. In mild to moderate cases, surgery to remove implants via laser, heat (cauterisation) or the knife is possible – either through a laparoscope or a cut in the abdomen. This can also remove cysts or adhesions. The more radical option is a hysterectomy, with or without removal of the ovaries. It is major surgery with major side effects, physically and psychologically, including a need for HRT (hormone replacement therapy) if the ovaries are removed. It is never a procedure to be entered into lightly and the decision should be yours and yours alone – not your doctor's or anyone else's.

Natural Alternatives

Conventional medical treatments do not suit all women. Some also find that their symptoms are not taken seriously by their doctor. There is a range of alternative therapies that you may prefer to try. Although there are no research figures to back them up, complementary therapists report a good success rate. But bear in mind that, like the drugs a doctor may prescribe, these remedies may not suit every woman.

- Homeopaths and herbalists claim that a combination of vitamin and mineral supplements can help reduce inflammation and boost the body's immune system, and that certain herbs can help to correct hormonal problems.

    They stress, however, that every woman must be treated as an individual and as a

whole – and that the results won't be immediate. But after three to six months, they should start to show – and can be very good. The treatment programme is likely to include a range of vitamin and mineral supplements (including special preparations of zinc and calcium), herbal tinctures, homeopathic remedies, flower essences, and advice on diet and lifestyle changes.
- Chinese medicine works well for some women, too. It's a combination of herbal therapy, dietary advice, acupuncture, massage and sometimes other techniques with their roots in the traditional Chinese system.

COMPLICATIONS

The bleeding and scarring associated with endometriosis can lead to what are called adhesions; these can be so widespread that they cause the pelvic organs to stick to one another. Another problem is the development of cysts. Some can grow quite large and are filled with dark, altered blood; these are known as chocolate cysts. Both conditions can cause fertility problems and pain.

Self-help

There are ways that you can help yourself, such as changing your diet, mineral supplements, and using techniques for pain management.

- **Painkillers:** Aspirin and paracetamol are both useful in relieving mild to moderate pain. Aspirin can be the more effective because it blocks production of prostaglandins, but you may also find that it has side effects such as stomach irritation or even bleeding. Remember, too, that analgesics only treat the symptom, not the endometriosis.
- **Vitamins and other supplements:** Some women have had success with vitamin B6 and evening primrose oil. Vitamin C also helps healing and can reduce heavy bleeding, and vitamin E is often recommended to prevent thick scar tissue forming.
- **Diet:** The emphasis is on low-fat, high-fibre foods, and preferably organic ones. Some complementary therapists believe there is a link between endometriosis and candida (the organism that causes thrush), so a diet avoiding sugar, yeast and refined or processed foods may be of benefit.
- **Heat:** The good old hotwater bottle, heating pad, hot bath or electric blanket can be a blessing.
- **Exercise:** If you are in chronic pain you may not feel like exercise, but not only can it improve your fitness, it can also increase production of those feel-good endorphins. But check with your doctor first and avoid any jarring activity, such as jogging, which could tug at adhesions and scar tissue. Swimming is good, as are aquarobics, Tai chi and yoga.

- **Relaxation:** You may have your own favourite way of winding down; deep breathing, muscle relaxation or visualisation can all work well, given time and practice.

> **IMPORTANT NOTE**
>
> Despite the distress and discomfort it causes, endometriosis is a benign disease. It is simply the growth of normal tissue in abnormal places — unlike cancer, which is the growth of abnormal tissue.

Chapter 8
Too Little, Too Much, Too Late
Or Not at All

Although the most common menstrual problems are period pain or PMS, there are a number of others – including **amenorrhoea** (failure to bleed), **menorrhagia** (heavy bleeding), **oligomenorrhoea** (infrequent, irregular periods) and **hypomenorrhoea** (scanty periods).

AMENORRHOEA

This is when your period fails to arrive, even though you are usually regular; less commonly, it means failure to menstruate at all. Most women suffer one or more episodes of amenorrhoea during their life. On the other hand, it affects 1 per cent of women from puberty – this is known as primary amenorrhoea.

These are the main causes:

- **Pregnancy:** This is by far the most usual reason! Amenorrhoea is also fairly common in the early stages of breastfeeding. But this doesn't mean you can forget about contraception; many a woman has found to her dismay that she has become pregnant again before her first period after the birth of a child.

- **Hormonal imbalance:** This can happen if there's a breakdown in the link between the hypothalamus, the pituitary gland and the ovaries. The most frequent causes of this are stress, or being very overweight or underweight (such as with the eating disorders anorexia nervosa and bulimia). Women who exercise a lot, such as high performance athletes or dancers, may also find their periods stop.
- **Tumour on pituitary gland:** This tumour prevents the pituitary gland sending out its chemical messengers, so the whole system grinds to a halt.
- **Post-pill:** Sometimes, and for no real reason, your system can be a bit sluggish after being on the pill, and may need a kick-start to stimulate the ovaries to work again.
- **Ovarian disease:** This could be caused by various conditions from endometriosis to multiple cysts, infection or cancer (see Chapter 9).
- **Premature menopause:** In the years leading up to menopause, your periods are likely to become irregular and may even stop altogether for months at a time. Although the average age for menopause is between 45 and 50, for some women it can come as early as 30.

- **Drug use:** If you take tranquillisers or narcotics, you may find your periods affected.
- **Chronic diseases:** Thyroid problems, anaemia and a number of other conditions can lead to menstrual failure.

With primary amenorrhoea, the causes may be:

- **Congenital abnormality:** This could involve the uterus, ovaries or tubes; in some cases, the organs may be missing.
- **Imperforate hymen:** This just means that the hymen is blocking the flow of blood; it's a condition easy to fix.
- **Chromosome abnormalities:** A rare condition.

Treatment

This depends on the cause of the problem. Here's a rundown of the most common:

- **Hormone therapy:** For hormonal imbalance, premature menopause, or post-pill sluggishness.
- **Lifestyle changes:** Weight gain if you're underweight, weight loss if you're overweight, cutting back on exercise or drug use.
- **Surgery:** For pituitary tumour, ovarian cysts, an imperforate hymen.
- **Herbal and homeopathic remedies:** Your complementary therapist will guide you, but remedies can include tansy tea.

- **Reassurance:** For many women, there may be no real cause and, if this is the case, it's important to realise that there's nothing harmful in not having your period – it almost always returns in time. Some women even find that they start bleeding soon after seeing the doctor or just making the appointment!

MENORRHAGIA

The causes of heavy bleeding can include:

- **Pathological conditions:** If you are over 35, the most likely cause is either polyps or fibroids (see Chapter 9). Infection may also be a possibility.
- **Miscarriage:** If you're a week or so late and the bleed is heavier than usual, get your doctor to check it out, as it could be an early miscarriage.
- **Anovulatory cycles:** Sometimes the bleeding is heavier in cycles in which you fail to ovulate.
- **IUD:** Some women with an IUD find their periods are often later and heavier than they were before they had it fitted.

Treatment

Medical treatment will depend on the cause. If the problem is hormonal imbalance, the heavy bleeding may clear up of its own accord after a couple of months. If not – and you are also showing signs of anaemia (tiredness, dizziness, pale skin, headaches) – your doctor may suggest putting you on the pill for a few months, or some other type of hormone such as progesterone.

If fibroids or polyps are to blame, surgery may be necessary as the condition is unlikely to clear spontaneously. You may also need surgery in the form of a D&C if a late, heavy bleed turns out to be a miscarriage – or antibiotics if an infection is to blame.

If the flooding is related to an IUD, your doctor may suggest that you consider some other form of contraception. Complementary therapies will also help some women – for instance, if the cause is hormonal imbalance – but the treatment will depend on the problem. But alas, there's little you can do for yourself.

OLIGOMENORRHOEA

There may be no 'cause' – it may simply be that your menstrual pattern is one in which your periods don't arrive every 28 days on schedule. On the other hand, it could be that your hormones are playing up – or slowing down, especially if you are near the age at which menopause is a possibility.

Treatment

Your doctor can arrange for a blood test that can throw more light on the situation. If it's simply a case of your body finding a pattern, no treatment will be necessary, but reassurance can put your mind at rest.

On the other hand, if you're premenopausal, hormone therapy of one form or other may be suitable. This could mean putting you on the pill, although this may mask what else may be happening to your body in the run-up to menopause; or hormone replacement therapy in which oestrogen is taken daily, and possibly progesterone too for a certain number of days each month. Of course, if you're not getting any other symptoms of menopause and the irregular bleeding doesn't bother you, the simplest solution could be just to do nothing.

HYPOMENORRHOEA

This is a long name for having light periods. The reasons may be:

- **Age:** Many women in their premenopausal years find their periods become scantier.
- **Weight loss or exercise:** The development of anorexia or bulimia or a stepped-up exercise programme can affect how much you bleed.
- **Hormonal imbalance:** If your hormones are out of whack, your periods may be lighter.

Treatment

Clearly, if the cause relates to something you are doing to your body – as in anorexia or heavy exercise – the treatment lies in changing your lifestyle, and both your doctor or a complementary therapist may be able to advise you.

Some women don't mind light periods – rather the reverse, so if the situation is a result of being premenopausal, no treatment may be required. If the hormone imbalance is not menopause-linked, hormone therapy, such as the pill, may be suggested. Natural remedies which work in the same way as your own hormones may also help; your complementary therapist can advise you.

Chapter 9
When the System Goes Wrong

There is a wide range of diseases and conditions that can affect the various parts of a woman's reproductive system, beyond those already discussed in the preceding chapters. It seems that no part of the reproductive system is immune from trouble! Some of these problems are more serious than others, and may include:

CERVIX

- **Cervical 'erosion':** This is something of a misleading term as it suggests that your cervix may be wearing away – this isn't the case. Neither is it an ulcer, as it's sometimes called. It's just a case of some of the mucus cells in the cervix poking out into the vagina. It's a minor condition, and little if any treatment is needed.
- **Cervical cancer:** This strikes 2 to 3 per cent of women, mainly between the ages of 25 and 55. It can be cured if caught early, but the chances drop to 50 per cent or less once the cancer becomes advanced.

That's why regular cervical smears are vital. Smears can pick up abnormalities in the cells (cervical dysplasia) that, if untreated, may lead to cancer.

If further tests show the early stages of cancer (carcinoma in situ), an operation called a cone biopsy can be carried out to remove the affected areas.

Where the cancer is advanced, a hysterectomy may be needed. If the cancer has spread, the ovaries may be removed along with other organs and radiation may also be necessary.

Cervical cancer is more likely in women who started sex early and have many sexual partners. There is also a link with the sexually transmitted disease, genital wart virus.

UTERUS

- **Uterine or endometrial cancer:** The only accurate way to diagnose this is by carrying out a D&C and examining the endometrial cells under a microscope. Most cases occur in women who have passed menopause, but about a quarter are in younger women. The symptoms include irregular or heavy bleeding, or vaginal discharge. Treatment normally involves a total hysterectomy. The ovaries also have to be removed because of the risk that the hormones they produce may trigger any endometrial cells still dormant. For this

reason, hormone replacement therapy can't be used either. If caught early, there's a good chance of recovery, but in advanced cases the outlook is poor.
- **Polyps:** These are smooth, fleshy, noncancerous growths that develop on a kind of stalk attached to the internal surface of either the uterus or the cervix. They can cause bleeding or discharge if they become eroded or infected, and can be removed surgically. If there are a number of polyps on the endometrium, they can be removed with a D&C.
- **Fibroids:** These are a different kind of non-cancerous growths, made up of muscle and fibrous tissues. It's estimated that about 20 per cent of women over 30 have fibroids, and often have no symptoms. But if you suffer painful, gushy, clotty bleeds, have backache or a sudden increase in the need to urinate, fibroids may be to blame. If they are causing no trouble, no treatment may be necessary and the fibroids generally shrink with menopause. Where they are a problem, surgery can be used to hollow out individual fibroids; another option may be a hysterectomy.

OVARIES

- **Cysts:** There's a whole range of cysts that can affect your ovaries. The most common are either **follicular** or **corpus luteum** cysts. Follicular cysts develop when, for some unknown reason, the follicle doesn't release the egg at ovulation; instead, it swells up with clear fluid and becomes a cyst. They often produce no symptoms and most disappear after a few menstrual cycles. Corpus luteum cysts develop when the corpus luteum does not shrink and die as it's supposed to do 14 or so days after ovulation. Like follicular cysts, they rarely get bigger than a large plum but can lead to hormone imbalance and irregular bleeding. They can rupture and may have to be removed surgically.

OVARIAN CYSTS

These include a couple of unpleasant-sounding ones; dermoid cysts, which can include hair and teeth; mucous cysts, jelly-like cysts that can grow to a whopping 14kg. Most cysts like these are harmless, but if they are large they can affect the blood supply to the ovaries and should be removed.

- **Cancer:** While it is less common than cancer of the uterus or cervix, ovarian cancer causes more deaths because it is often not detected until the late stages. It occurs mainly in women over 50, and those who are childless or have a fertility problem. Early symptoms may be little more than vague discomfort, and it is hard to pick up abnormalities with a physical examination as the ovaries are deep within the pelvis; an ultrasound is the most reliable way. In the early stages, it may be possible just to remove the affected ovary. But in most cases, treatment involves taking out both ovaries, the Fallopian tubes and any other organs to which the cancer has spread. This may be combined with anticancer drugs and radiation.

OTHER CANCERS

- **Vulva:** This accounts for only about 3 per cent of all pelvic cancers.
- **Vagina:** This makes up about 1 per cent of pelvic cancers, mostly in women over 55.
- **Fallopian tubes:** This is a very rare condition which affects mainly older women.

CERVICAL SMEARS

Developed more than half a century ago by Dr George Papanicolaou, these have probably saved the lives of thousands, if not millions of women. Cells are collected from the cervix using a wooden spatula and/or cyto brush, and examined under the microscope. It is recommended that you have a cervical smear every 3 years — especially after the age of 25.

Helpful Addresses

There are a range of organisations that can lend practical advice and support to those who suffer from problems associated with periods. The head offices of support groups listed may be able to put you in touch with a local branch in your area. Meeting and talking to those with similar problems can be very helpful. The professional organisations listed may be able to advise you on how to find a complementary therapist.

National Association for Premenstrual Syndrome (NAPS)
PO Box 72
Sevenoaks
Kent
TN13 1XG
(01732) 741709

British Homeopathic Association
27A Devonshire Street
London
W1N 1RJ
(0171) 735 2163

British Naturopathic and Osteopathic Association
Frazer House
6 Netherhall Gardens
London
NW3 5RR

Endometriosis Society
Unit 7A
8 Shakespeare Business Centre
245A Coldharbour Lane
London
SW9 8RR
(0171) 737 0380

Family Planning Association
27–35 Mortimer Street
London
W1N 7RJ
(0171) 636 7866

Institute of Complementary Medicine
PO Box 194
London
SE16 1QZ
(0171) 237 5165

International Stress Management Association
The Priory Hospital
Priory Lane
London
SW15 5JJ
(01532) 664260

Self-Help in Pain (SHIP)
33 Kingsdown Park
Tankerton
Kent
CT5 2DT
(01227) 264677

TENS Unit
Spembly Medical Company Ltd
Newbury Road
Andover
Hants
SP10 4DR
(01264) 365741

Women's Therapy Centre
6 Manor Gardens
London
N7 6LA
(0171) 263 6200

Glossary

Adhesions: bands of scar tissue; can bind organs together
Amenorrhoea: absence of menstruation
Analgesics: painkillers
Anovulatory: a cycle in which ovulation does not occur
Anti-prostaglandin: an agent that blocks or reduces production of prostaglandins
Beta-sympathomimetics: drugs that mimic the effect of adrenalin and act on the smooth muscles of the body, such as the uterus; used occasionally to stop cramping
Carcinoma in situ: the very early stages of cervical cancer
Cervical canal: canal linking the cervix to the main part of the uterus
Cervical cancer: cancer of the cervix
Cervical dysplasia: changes in cervical cells that may be a precursor to cancer
Cervical erosion: this occurs when mucus cells from the cervical canal pout out into the vagina; these may become red and infected, possibly causing bleeding or discharge

Cervical os: the tiny opening in the cervix

Cervical smear: a procedure in which cells are scraped gently from the cervix and checked under a microscope for signs of abnormalities and/or cervical cancer

Cervix: the neck of the womb

Chocolate cyst: endometrial cyst full of dark, thick blood

Clitoris: a pink, exquisitely sensitive knob-like protruberance located just below where the labia minora meet

Corpus luteum: remains of the follicle after ovulation; produces progesterone in second part of the menstrual cycle

Cyst: an enclosed swelling, usually full of fluid or mucus

D&C: dilation and curettage of the uterus, in which the endometrium is scraped out

Dysmenorrhoea: period pain

Dyspareunia: pain during intercourse

Ectopic pregnancy: a pregnancy in which the fertilised egg implants outside the uterus, often in the Fallopian tube

Endometriosis: a condition in which endometrial cells are found attached to organs other than the uterus

Endometrium: the cells lining the inside of the uterus

Evening primrose oil: an extract high in vitamin E, an essential fatty acid (gammalinoleic acid) used in the treatment of a number of menstrual problems

Fallopian tube: tube through which the newly-released egg travels from the ovary to the uterus

Fibroid: noncancerous tumour made up of fibre or muscle tissue that develops within the uterus or uterine walls

Follicle: small sac in which the egg develops within the uterus

FSH: Follicle stimulating hormone, a chemical messenger sent by the pituitary gland to prompt ripening of the egg within the follicle

GnRH: gonadotropin-releasing hormone sometimes used to treat endometriosis

HRT: hormone replacement therapy

Hypomenorrhoea: very light menstruation

Hypothalamus: the part of the brain that controls the pituitary gland

Hysterectomy: surgical removal of the uterus; a total hysterectomy involves removal of the ovaries and possibly the Fallopian tubes, too

IUD: intrauterine device used for contraception

Labia majora: the outer lips of the vulva

Labia minora: the inner lips of the vulva

Laparoscopy: a small operation in which the abdominal cavity and organs are viewed by using a small telescope-like instrument known as a laparoscope, inserted via a small cut usually in the area of the navel

LH: luteinising hormone, produced by the pituitary gland to prompt ovulation and production of progesterone by the corpus luteum

LHRH: luteinising hormone-releasing hormone

Menarche: the onset of menstruation

Menopause: the cessation of menstruation
Menorrhagia: excessive blood loss during menstruation
Menstruation: the period, a flow of blood and endometrial tissue from the uterus signalling the end of one menstrual cycle and the start of the next
Mittelschmerz: pain on ovulation
Monophasic pill: type of contraceptive pill in which the levels of oestrogen and progesterone remain the same
Oestrogen: female sex hormone produced by the ovaries
Oligomenorrhoea: irregular periods
Ovary: the female sex organ in which seed eggs are stored and developed
Ovulation: the release of the mature egg from the ovary
PID: pelvic inflammatory disease
Pituitary gland: the gland located at the base of the brain, under the command of the hypothalamus, which releases chemical messengers such as follicle stimulating hormone and luteinising hormone
Polyps: noncancerous fleshy growths that develop on stalk-like protuberances
Premenstruum: the phase of the cycle between ovulation and the start of your period, often referring specifically to the three or four days before the onset of bleeding
PMS: premenstrual syndrome, a variety of physical, psychological and emotional symptoms relating to the premenstrual phase

Pre-sacral neurectomy: a surgical procedure in which the nerves that transmit pain from the uterus to the brain are cut

Progesterone: female sex hormone produced by the corpus luteum

Prolactin: a female hormone that helps ovulation

Prostaglandins: short-lived substances produced throughout the body to control the function of smooth muscles such as the uterus

Retrograde menstruation: a backwash of blood and endometrial cells

Retroverted uterus: a uterus that tips backwards instead of forwards

TENS: transcutaneous electrical nerve stimulation, a device used in pain management to block pain messages to the brain

Testosterone: a male sex hormone

Triphasic pill: a type of contraceptive pill in which the levels of oestrogen and progesterone vary in parts of the cycle

Urethra: opening of the urinary tract

Uterus: (womb) hollow, muscular pear-shaped organ lined by the endometrium and which houses the developing foetus

Vagina: muscular-walled canal connecting the cervix to the vulva

Vitamin B6: also known as pyridoxine, a vitamin found useful in treating various menstrual disorders

Vulva: the female genital area

Robinson Family Health

All your health questions answered in a way you really understand

Available from leading bookshops, or from Robinson using the order form below
or by writing to the address given

ORDER FORM

Please Tick

Arthritis: What Really Works
Dava Sobel & Arthur C Klein £7.99
"I cannot recommend this book too highly."
Dr James Le Fanu, Daily Telegraph

☐

Asthma: Breathe Easy
Megan Gressor £2.99

☐

Brain Damage: Don't Learn to Live With It!
Margaret Baker and Trevor England £7.99

☐

Bulima Nervosa & Binge Eating
Dr Peter Cooper £6.99
"Highly recommended." British Journal of Psychiatry

☐

The Good Diet Guide: Choose the diet that's right for you
Dr Jane Dunkeld £6.99

☐

Headaches: Relief at Last
Megan Gressor £2.99

☐

Massage for Common Ailments
Penny Rich £4.99 (full colour)

☐

Overcoming IBS
Dr Christine P Dancey and Susan Backhouse £6.99
"A simply excellent book" Dr James Le Fanu, Sunday Telegraph

☐

Practical Aromatherapy
Penny Rich £4.99 (full colour)

☐

The Recovery Book: A Life-saving Guide for Alcoholics and Addicts
Al J Mooney, A & H Eisenburg £9.99
"The most complete and accurate compendium I've ever read."
James W West, Betty Ford Centre

☐

Women's Waterworks: Curing Incontinence
Pauline Chiarelli £2.99

☐

You *Can* Beat Period Pain
Liz Kelly £2.99

☐

Orders to: Robinson Publishing Ltd., 7 Kensington Church Court, London W8 4SP

I enclose a cheque for £ _____ in payment for the books indicated above.
Post & Packing FREE within the UK, please add 20% for postage outside the UK.

Name: _____

Address: _____

_____ Postcode: _____

(Please allow 28 days for delivery in the UK, longer elsewhere)

☐ Tick here if you would like to receive information on new health titles from Robinson